Cosmetic and Domestic Uses of Herbs

Making Your Own Natural Herbal Products

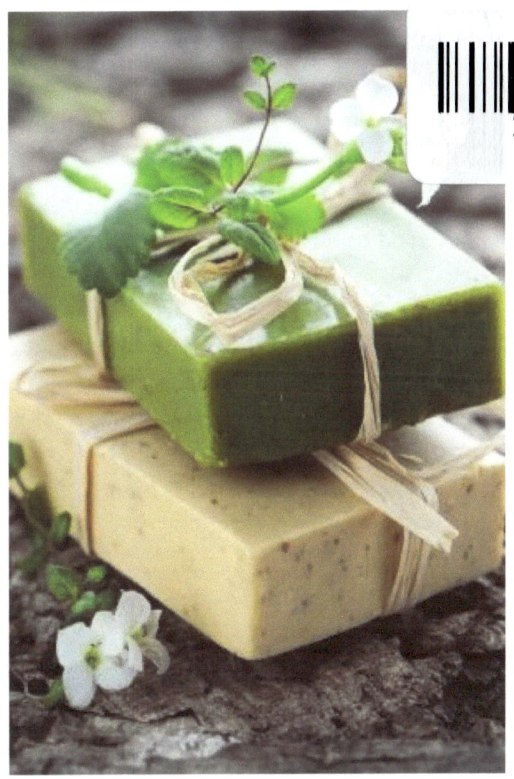

Dueep Jyot Singh

Healthy Learning Series

Mendon Cottage Books

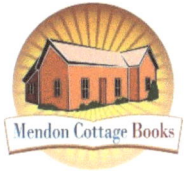

JD-Biz Publishing

All Rights Reserved.

No part of this publication may be reproduced in any form or by any means, including scanning, photocopying, or otherwise without prior written permission from JD-Biz Corp Copyright © 2016

All Images Licensed by Fotolia and 123RF.

Disclaimer

The information is this book is provided for informational purposes only. The information is believed to be accurate as presented based on research by the author.

The author or publisher is not responsible for the use or safety of any procedure or treatment mentioned in this book. The author or publisher is not responsible for errors or omissions that may exist.

Our books are available at

1. Amazon.com
2. Barnes and Noble
3. Itunes
4. Kobo
5. Smashwords
6. Google Play Books

Download Free Books!

http://MendonCottageBooks.com

Table of Contents

Introduction

When I began writing about the products you could make, at home, and sell from home, in your own small business, I had not thought about the multitude of uses, man has found for plants. For millenniums he has used herbs and parts of plants for culinary, medicinal, and domestic purposes.

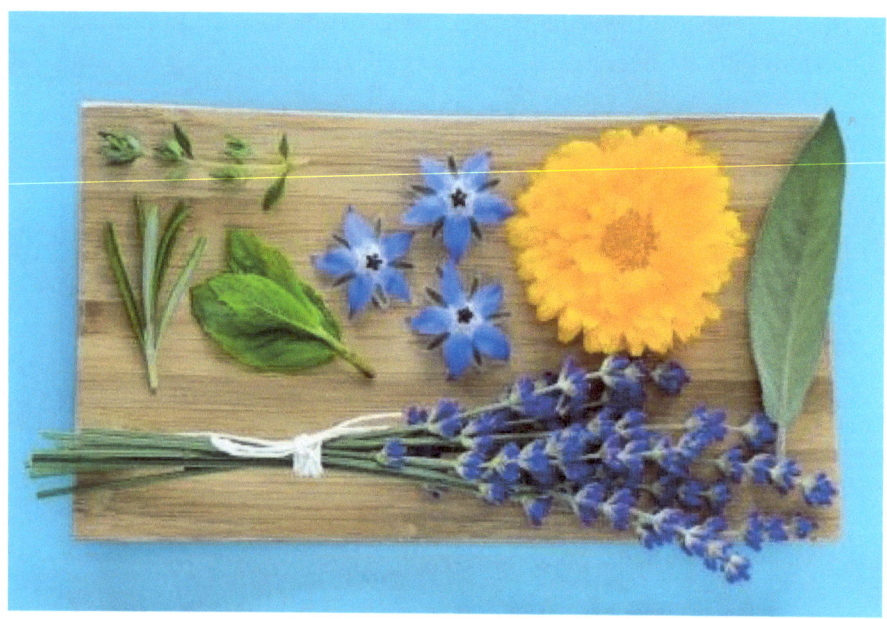

Apart from the well-known traditional use for all manners of illnesses and ailments – I defy any person in the world who has not used some natural cure, natural remedy, or even natural beauty recipe in order to cure himself naturally, – herbs have also proven to be invaluable in many other different ways, when you take it in the domestic context.

For centuries men have been using plants to provide shelter, fire material, floor coverings, roof coverings, and even utensils. Even today, in many parts of the world, the calabash is hollowed out and used as a container to store water as well as food. I have often used half of coconut shells in order to drink water, whenever I have gone trekking. Apart from this, herbs and plants have been used to provide color, decoration, flavor, and healthy benefits to a large number of our culinary preparations.

This book is going to tell you how you can use natural herbs and plants to create a large number of products, that you can either sell outside in your neighborhood, city, or use at home. Many of these methods have been time-tested and have been used down the ages to provide us with useful items, even though we have half forgotten about how to make them, because it is so easy for us to get them off the supermarket shelf.

Nevertheless, even if you do not use this book for providing you with items for sale, you can use it as a ready reference whenever you want to practice creating something naturally, profitably, and beneficial.

Let us just go into the woods. Many of us do not know that grasses, reeds, straw, leaves, branches, Heather, and turf have been used extensively down the ages to provide man with roof shelter, so if you do find yourself in a situation when you need to make a shelter to protect yourself from the elements start collecting these materials. After that, you are going to clean out your shelter with a number of birch twigs, which are still used as brooms. Incidentally, brooms are also called besoms, and that is why if you call a woman a besom, you are calling her a witch in any other way, because of her association with a broomstick! Heather is also an excellent broom. Naturally, the broom plant got its name from its domestic use.

Now we come to Birch bark. I was reading a JT Etson where Calamity Jane showing off as usual, fashioned household trays from birchbark. This bark was stretched into shape, and then allowed to dry. The Native Americans have been using this method to make household utensils for centuries.

https://www.youtube.com/watch?v=xL2lEqDnvLw is fascinating.

Thanks to the silica content coming down from prehistoric times in horsetails, they have been used as excellent scouring materials, especially for pots and pans, due to their abrasive qualities. This mineral is present in the stalks of Dutch Rush – also known as the scouring rush or pewter wart, equisetum hyemale is its scientific name. You can use it to clean pewter, saucepans, baking utensils, and any wooden kitchen surfaces. After all, this has been done down the centuries effectively.

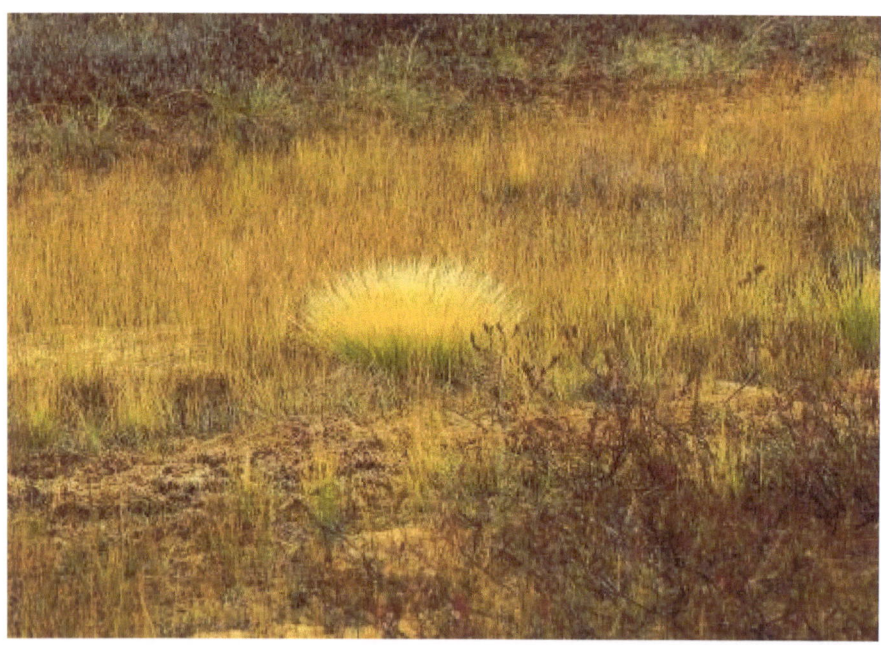

Dutch Rush

You can also use it as a polishing material because of the abrasive silica. Just tie a number of horsetails together and you are going to get an effective whisk in the preparation of washing materials.

Make sure that you do not use the dried plant, because it is going to fall off the stem. You can also use plants with a high acid content like rhubarb or sorrel, boiled with water to make a paste and apply it on the surface to give it a high-gloss. However, do not leave this paste on for a long while on aluminum utensils because it is capable of burning a hole.

Uses of Soapwort

This is one often overlooked herb, which was used extensively in ancient times, but with the coming of chemical-based cleaners and cosmetics, Saponaria officianalis's cleansing qualities are slowly being forgotten. When I was young, my grandmother used to put two handfuls of dried soapwort seeds into a bucket full of water, and leave it overnight. In the morning, she used it to wash our woolen clothes in it, as a mild detergent, which managed to get rid off all the dirt without harming that delicate fabric.

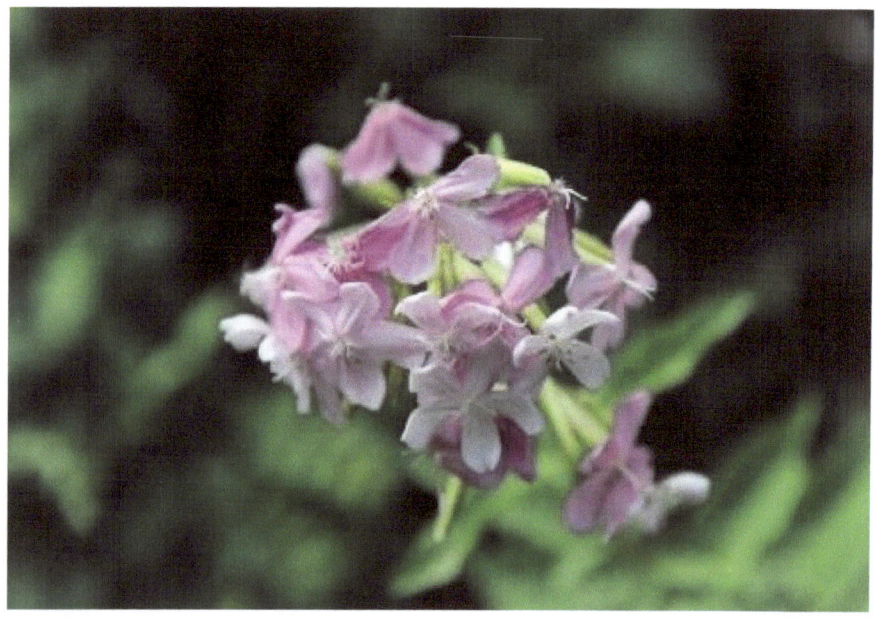

Soapwart

It is also called latherwort. Also, if you have some leaves at hand, make a decoction of it in boiling water. You just put in three handfuls of these leaves, and water and allow to boil untilthe quantity has been reduced. This green liquid is extremely good, to preserve old fibers, especially those which have been dyed to their original brightness. The green coloration is going to wash out in the rinsing. Professionals use this when they are restoring valuable silks, brocades, and tapestries in museums.

Pomanders and Air Fresheners

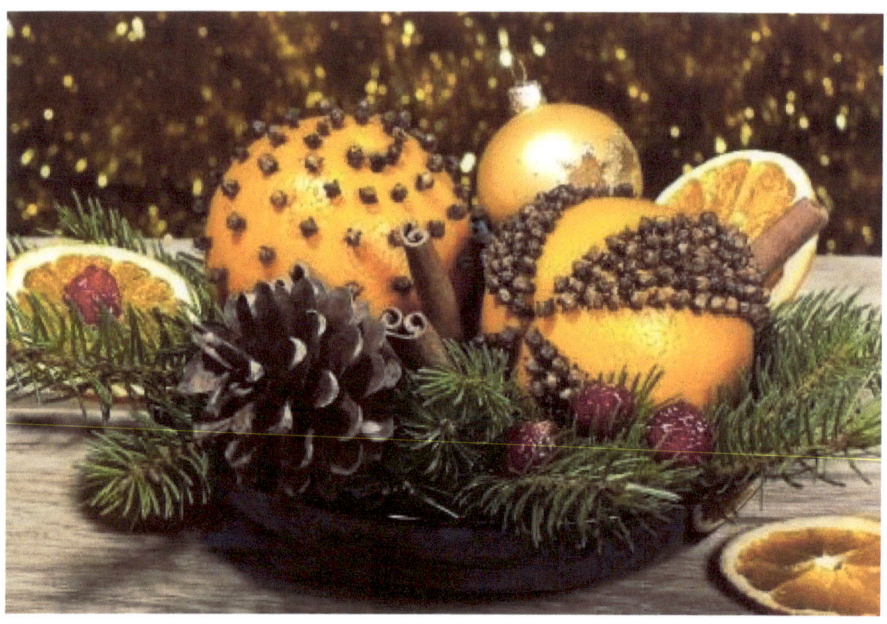

In medieval times, especially when people did not bother much about personal hygiene, they were quite adept at making air fresheners and pomanders, which they hung amidst their clothes either on their bodies, or in their wardrobes. Naturally, only a few rich people who could afford the money to buy cloves and oranges. Many just walked by on the streets, smelling and sniffing their pomanders. These are extremely easy to prepare, and you can leave them hanging either as Christmas decorations on Christmas trees, or in your wardrobe. For this, you are going to use thin-skinned fruit, especially citrus fruits like oranges, so that the punctures in the fruits' skin allows the essential oil to be set free. You can also use lemons and instead of cloves, you can also use aromatic seeds like cumin and fennel. You can either cut the skin or you can make small, shallow holes in the peel not deep enough to pierce the flesh. Put the cloves in the holes either in rows or in patches or at random. Finish by rubbing the pomander with ground cloves and salt and hang, with a ribbon, which you have wound through one cut, which goes all around the orange, and just deep enough to hold the ribbon.

You can dry the orange for a day or two above the stove in your kitchen, and after that, you can push the cloves into the entire surface of the skin so that just the heads peep out. The Elizabethans used bodkins to make the holes. You can also make the finishing powder like they did with equal amounts of cinnamon powder and orris powder and leave the orange wrapped in this mixture for the next two weeks. After that, they shook out the excess powder after unwrapping the fruit, tied a colorful silk ribbon around the groove and used while mincing down the smelly dirty roads. You can also hang this up and allow to dry naturally in an airing cupboard.

Lavender Scented Beads

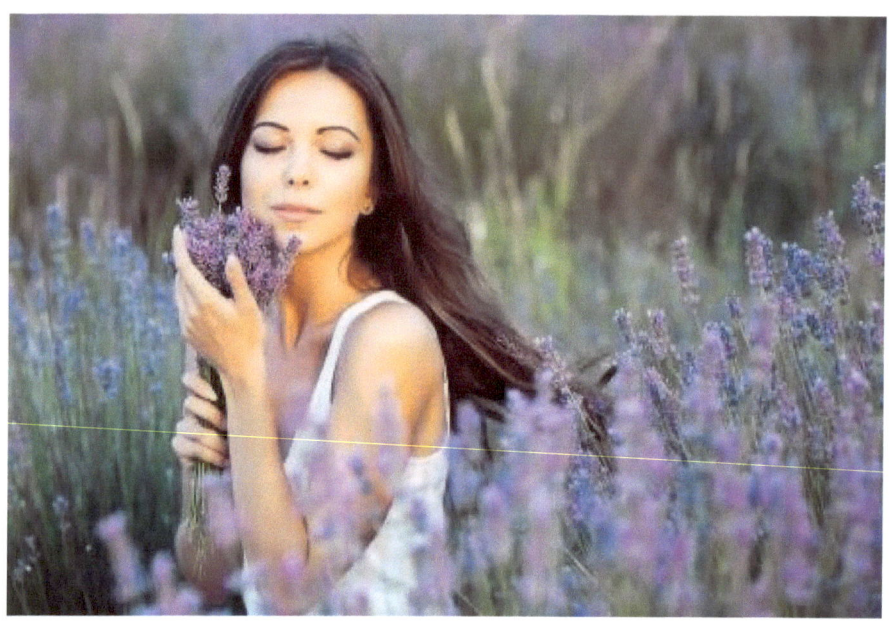

Lavender has a delicious scent

This is something I saw being sold extensively in a number of exhibitions, and they are so popular, this is how you make them. Just take three level tablespoons full of dried lavender flowers, 2 tablespoons full of sandalwood powder, one teaspoonful of powdered gum tragacanth, three drops essence of ambergris, lavender oil, 8 teaspoons full of orange flower water, one tablespoonful of gum benzoin, one tablespoonful of sweet flag root powder (Acorus calamus), one tablespoonful of orris root, and six drops of essence of lavender.

Like I said before, in medieval times up to the Victorian times, people made these sweet smelling items not only to ward off the terrible smells, but also to ward off the supposed diseases which were polluting the air.

Grind the flowers to a fine powder, and sift into a bowl with sweet flag root, sandalwood, and orris root powders. Add the gum benzoin and after that add the essences and ambergris.

Now you are going to dip your fingers in the mucilage which you have made up of gum tragacanth – 1 teaspoon with 8 teaspoons full of orange flower water. This mucilage is going to be used, to turn the powder into a paste. If the paste is not formed easily, add some more orange flower water.

Moisten your hands with some lavender oil and break the paste into small round beads. Roll each bead into the shape you like, round, oval, or any other shape. Pierce with a large needle and string immediately or place in a dark cupboard to dry, so that you can string them later. Remember to pierce, beforehand if you are drying them.

Air Sweeteners

Smudge Sticks and air fresheners are normally made by a number of aromatic herbs, especially evergreens like Juniper, sweet rushes, lavender, Tansy , etc., which were traditionally strewn on the ground to keep the atmosphere sweet smelling, and a floor covering, for all the stuff which fell down and was not snapped up by the dogs.

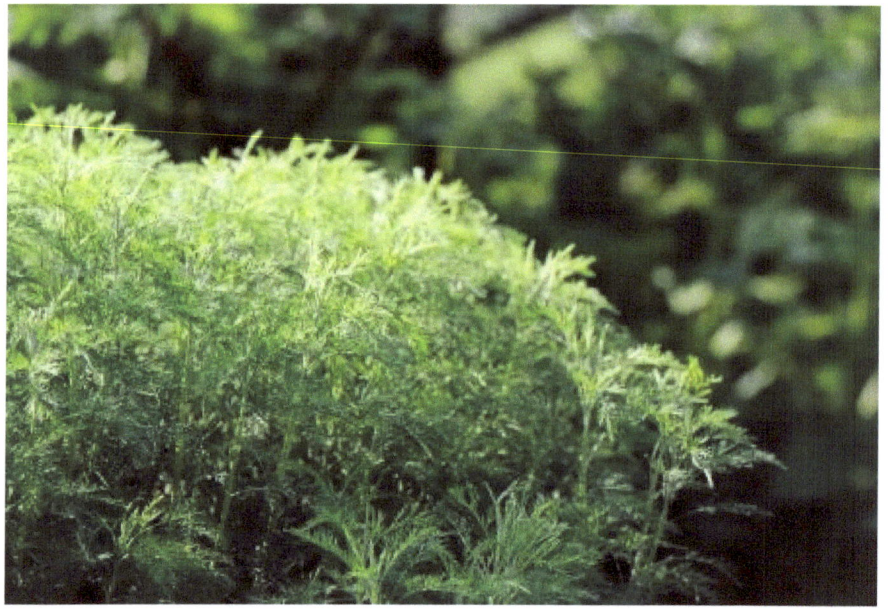

Artemisia

I was reading about a feast in ancient times, when the woman of the house made all her helping hands get rid of all the old rushes on the ground and strewed the ground with fresh herbs and grasses. You can use sweet Woodruff scattered behind books to get rid of the mustiness while you can also make pomanders, lavender bags, and nose gays of herbs like Penny Royal and Southern Wood.

Let us start with smudge sticks. If you find the natural incense burning in an Eastern Temple, or oriental home, well that is the traditional method in which people got rid of the smells and the humid and fetid atmosphere in a closed house, especially during the summer. If you want to fumigate your system, just make a traditional smoke inhalation mixture with one part fennel seeds, three parts sage, and one part aniseed. Crush the seeds gently so that the aromatic oils are expelled. Now mix them up with the sage leaves.

Put a small heap of this mixture on a fire, barbecue or hot coals. This is useful in asthma, or just infections, especially in children will have difficulty breathing. You are going to inhale the smoke with each intake, and when you exhale, you are going to expel your breath and fan the embers, if you have sprinkled the seeds on charcoal.

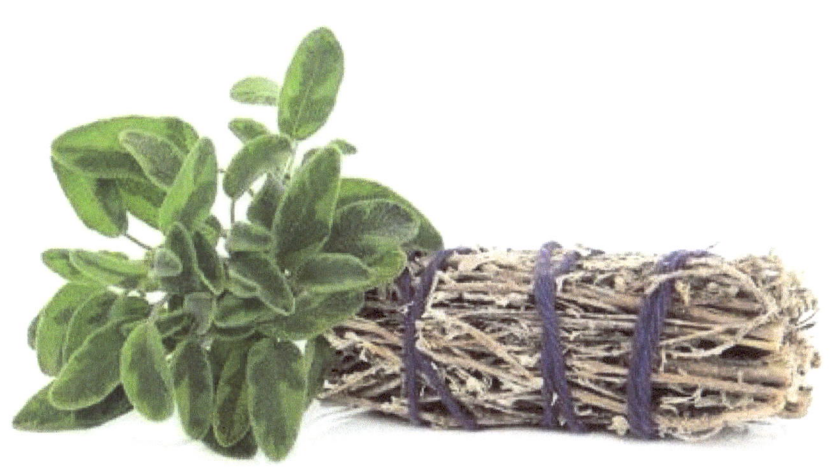

I normally use a small earthenware lamp because after all, I need a natural container in which to place the seeds. Then I set it alight and inhale the smoke to clear up my sinus problem.

Since ancient times, smudge sticks were used extensively to bring the fresh fragrance of nature into your house. Make up a bundle with sprigs of thyme, sage, rosemary, pine, cypress, fennel leaves, and stalks, and any other sweet smelling herbs you have around. Holding the sprigs together, tie them up in a tight bundled with a little bit of cotton thread. Do not use synthetic threads because they are going to smolder and fall off. After you have left the thread around the bundle to hold all the leaves in, tie securely every ½ inches and allow to dry naturally in a cool dry cupboard. After a couple of weeks, just hold the end of the smudge leaves, 2 inches above a candle flame. It is going to take a little while, but the end is going to become red and smolder releasing a trail of fragrant smoke. Some of the oily herbs/conifers, it may splutter and spit oil, especially if you are using Juniper. Once you feel that the air has been freshened enough, put your smudge sticks out carefully and trim the ends so they are ready for use the next time.

Making Aromatic Candles

These are also an excellent best-selling choice, in do-it-yourself exhibitions. See if you can get some good quality tallow and candle wax from a local craft shop. Marrow bone grease and beef fat tallow is also excellent, after you have boiled it well and filtered it. Incidentally, ancestors used to use animal fat in order to make natural cosmetics, and that is why I was looking at an old hair growing remedy, which spoke about some herbs melted in any animal fat, including puppy dog fat. Incidentally, this was a recipe taken from a 16 century Elizabethan recipe book, where they did not mind killing puppies for fat, while our 21st-century sensibilities shudder collectively at this idea.

Nevertheless, get some beef fat and tallow. Then collect some soft rushes, *Juncus conglomeratus,* which grow extensively in bogs, damp woodland, and wet pastures. For millenniums people have been using rush lights as the most economical source of domestic lighting and even now, in many rural areas, these rushes are used by gathering them, soaking for a few hours, and then allowed to dry outdoors in the sunshine. The outer husk is then stripped away, keep enough of the pithy part, and allowed to dry. This pith is then dipped **a number of times, and allowed to dry and then dipped again** in melted mutton fat, if you want to use them as rush lights. One rush light is capable of burning for half an hour giving you a soft light.

When you are using these reeds as candles, you have to secure them safely because they are not as stable as ordinary wax candles, even though you do not have to worry about dripping wax. Also they are longer in length. You can put them in special containers, so that you can keep shifting them as they burn. These are going to burn up to one hour indoors.

Herb Pillows and Lavender Bags

The first time I learned about herb pillows was when my grandmother who did not know that I was a chronic insomniac decided that a child which kept waking up with the roosters was not getting proper and adequate rest. And that is why she made a herb pillow for me. These are usually very small and like cushions. They did not solve my insomnia problem, then, because I spent the whole night sniffing the aroma while opening the window, looking at the moon, and doing everything else except sleeping, but seriously speaking, every sensible and normal person out there is going to go right off to sleep with these herbal pillows.

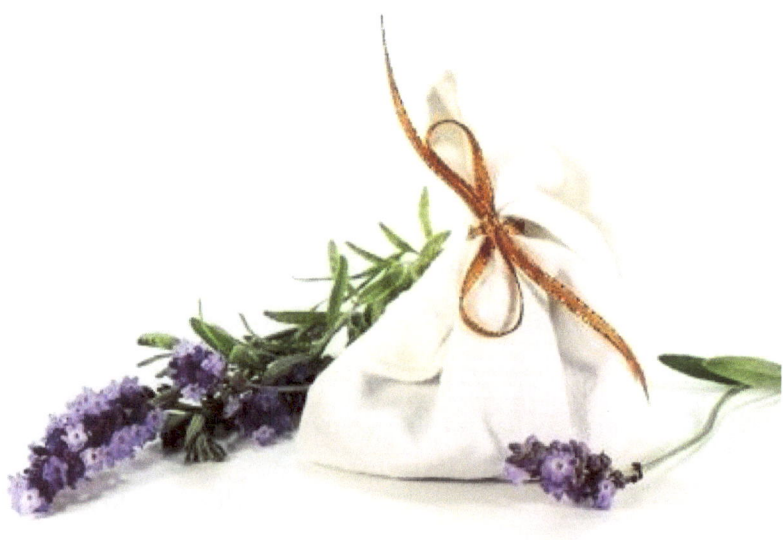

You may try this out as a neck rest. You can also use this as a charming gift, especially when you trim it with lace and ribbons.

In ancient times, dried hops were used extensively, to promote sleep. The Romans did it, but they made sure that the hops were replaced every four – six months after which they lost their strength.

Along with that, herb pillows also have dried petals, flower heads, and aromatic leaves, my grandmother added some powdered spices like cinnamon, sandalwood powder, orris root, lavender, rosemary, lemon Verbena, rose geranium, geranium, jasmine, rose flowers and rose leaves, and marjoram. The scents were enhanced with ground citrus orange peel and just one – two drops of essential aromatic oil like lavender, patchouli, and Neroli.

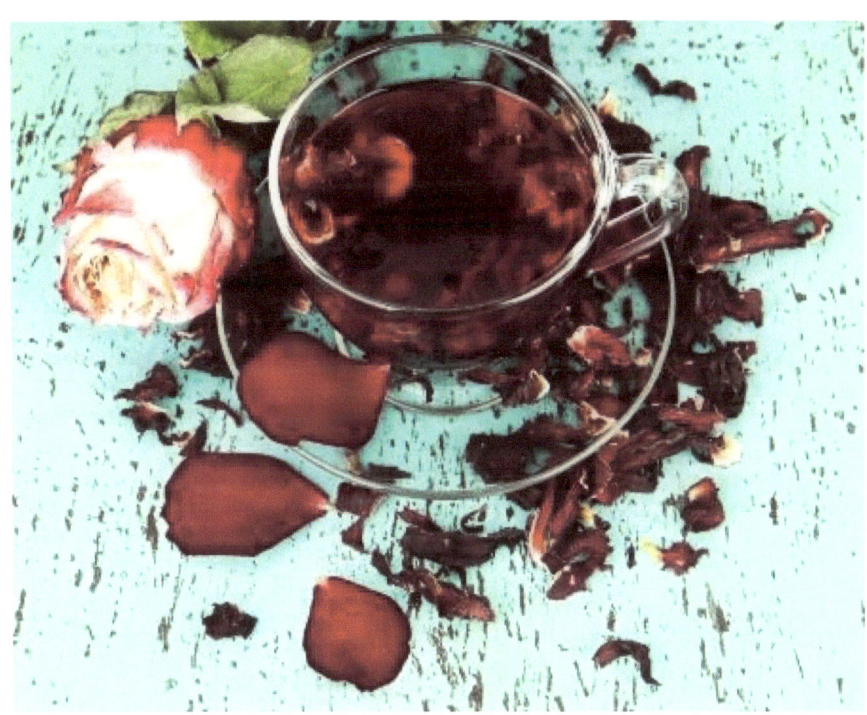

Herb Pillow Cover

The length and the width is going to depend upon the size of the pillow.

Back portion

0 – 1 and 2 – 3 is the total length of the pillow with one inch extra for seam allowance.

0 – 2 and 1 – 3 is the total width of the pillow +1 inch extra for seam allowance.

Draw rectangle by joining 0 – 1 – 2 – 3 and cut.

Front portion

Place the back part of the fabric and draw the outline. After that, remove the part because now you are going to mark an extension.

0 – 4, 0 – 5, 1 – 6, 1 – 7, 2 – 8, 2 – 9, 3 – 10 and 3 – 11 are marked all around. These are equal to double of the corner fold measurement.

That means if the corner fold is ½ inch because it is a small pillow, then you are going to take the measurement as one inch plus half an inch extra. Join all the corners with an extended outline, as seen in the figure below. 12, 13, 14 and 15 are the corner points. Join 4 – 5, 6 – 7, 8 – 9 and 10 – 11. Cut these corners for folding and stitching. Mark, draw, as shown in the figure, and cut.

The inner portion of the back is 0 – 1 and 2 – 3 =2 inches in length. 0 – 2, and 1 – 3 is going to be equal in width. Mark, draw, and cut.

How to sew

Bring together [fold] one edge of the back portion, and stitch with either 0 – 2 or 1 – 3 of the back inner portion. Match the corners of 4 – 5, 6 – 7, 8 – 9 and 10 – 11 and stitch on the wrong side. Press the seam and fold the corners. Now spread the front part of the pillow on the table by keeping the wrong side up facing you. Now place one side of the inner part on it by matching the unstitched edge of 0 – 2.

Place the back portion over this by matching 1 – 3 together, and for the corners of the 4, 6, 7, 11, 10, 8, 9 and 5. Fix with bead headed needles to keep in place, machine with a single stitch and after that you can use any sort of embroidery stitches like a closed zigzag stitch on the previous single plain stitch.

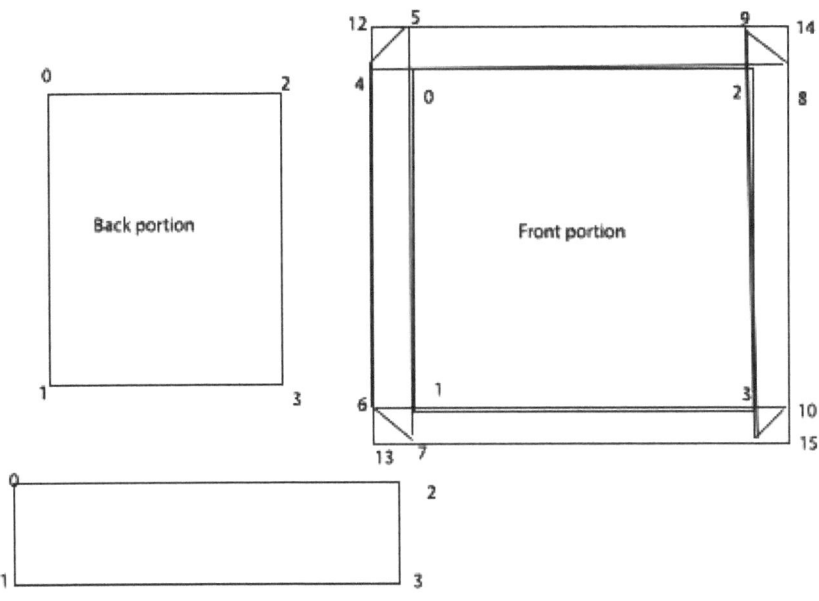

Once your pillowcase cover is made, it is easy to fill it up with a mixture of dried flowers and spices, given above, but I am giving you the recipe for a rosemary herb pillow. Take 4 cups of dried rosemary leaves and to that add 1 cup each of dried lemon verbena leaves, and 1 cup of dried pine needles. To this, you are going to add 1 tablespoon full of crushed orris root and two crushed cloves.

When you are adding the pine needles to this mixture make sure that the pillow slip is made up of really strong cotton fabric which has been closely woven, because these needles have a tendency of pricking out from their coverings.

You can also make a fragrant herb pillow by mixing together one cup each of dried rose petals, dried lavender, dried lemon verbena leaves, dried rosemary flowers and leaves, and any other dried flowers which you have, including carnations, geraniums, honeysuckle, lily of the valley, I like Jasmine, etc. You are going to fix the essential oils by adding the ground citrus lemon peel of 2 lemons and one orange or you can use an alternative of 2 teaspoons full of powdered Orris, or Sweet flag root or 3 drops of bergamot oil.

Sachet Bag with Dried Herbs

Keep this mixture at hand to stuff in sachet bags.

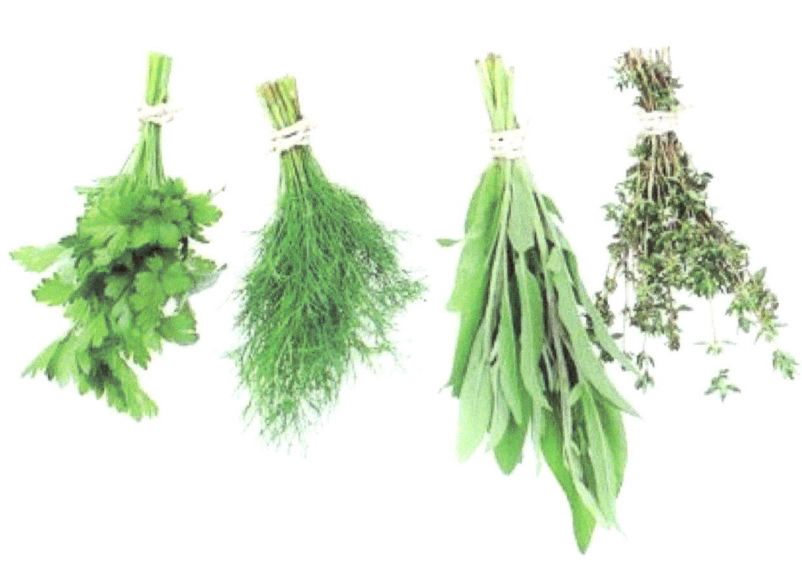

But before that, I am going to teach you how to dry herbs. Snip the herbs at the base of the stem with a pair of sharp scissors. Once you have gathered enough of these herbs, either put them in a paper bag or wrap them up in a kitchen towel and leave to dry in a warm dark well ventilated room for at least 2 days. If you have an airing cupboard so much the better. These herbs are ready for use, when they feel dry and are crumbly when you touch them. Once dried, crumbled them up into an tight container for storage purposes. After that you can use them either as herbal tea infusions, or in your cooking and also for the herb sweet smelling bags, I am telling you about.

There is one good thing about these herbal bags. These small scented bags are excellent to repel moths, while they keep our clothes smelling sweet. You will need just one little handful for one sachet bag and these can include dried herbs and spices. You can also use essential oils such as rosemary, lavender, cloves, mint, and thyme. In fact, if anything smells good and really strong and nice, you are going to use it in your bag. You can also use cinnamon sticks, dried citrus, and lemon peel, lavender oil, especially when you are making moth repellent bags and sleepy pillows.

For this, you just need 2 small squares of fabric, 10 cm into 10 cm of closely woven cotton, calico, or linen. Line up the 2 squares, with the right sides facing together – that means the wrong side is facing you – and sew around 3 of the 4 edges, either by hand or by a machine using a straight stitch and a 1 cm seam allowance. The 4th seam is left open for filling purposes. Now turn the bag right side out, and work out the corners with something sharp like a knitting needle. If you want to do any sort of decoration like adding a little bit of appliqué, or ribbon, you can do it on one of the squares, before you begin to sew.

Fill the bag up with your dried herb mixture which you have already crumbled and stripped of any stalks or sharp and bulky portions before hand. These herb petals and leaves are put in any bowl with spices and essential oils you like. You can also use dried flowers for bulk purposes. Now tuck in the final seam and sew. You could also gather together and tie it shut with a piece of ribbon and trim the edges with pinking shears.

These bags are capable of smelling sweet for about a year and whenever you think that the aroma is getting faint, all you have to do is sprinkle a few drops of some lavender or any other essential oil onto the fabric bag.

Moth Bag

A really effective moth bag can be made by mixing up equal quantities of dry lavender leaves with dried Tansy and Costmary leaves – *chrysanthemum balsamita*. Just mix them together in a pestle and mortar. Put them in a bag and this is going to be quite effective for the next 6 months. With a little bit of chrysanthemum cinerariifolium – also known as Pyrethrum, flowers and leaves, you are going to get an even more powerful moth bag.

Making Natural Gums and Glues

When I was small, and all the neighborhood children used to get together for amateur theatricals, we used to make our own costumes with jewelry and crowns cut out of cardboard, and sprinkled lavishly with golden dust, powder, artificial stones, and anything which glittered including sequins, spangles, pieces of golden thread, and whatever we could find. These were stuck together with starch, which was made by boiling a mixture of water and refined flour. Even today, this starch is used for starching clothes and for sticking purposes. So if you have gum Arabic *Acacia Senegal*, gum tragacanth *Astragalus gummifer,* or Carob gum (Ceratonia siliqua) you can make up a paste with powdered gum, and water in the proportions you require. Half a teaspoonful of gum is sufficient for half a cup of water.

Natural mucilage can be found in mistletoe berries, – have not you seen them really sticky, no wonder the word viscous comes from the scientific term for mistletoe Viscum album – and the bulbs of the bluebell. In the same way Holly gives you birdlime, which was used to catch small birds 500 years ago and even today, small birds are still caught in many parts of Europe with this birdlime.

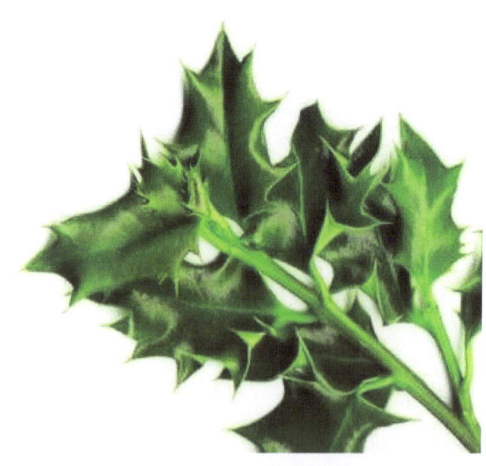

The bark of the Holly is stripped while it is still young. It is then soaked and boiled and then the inner layer is allowed to ferment in a closed container, which was sometimes buried. This produced mucilage which was then ground up and washed, and then fermented again. After that, it was mixed with the sticky substance to get an extremely sticky birdlime paste. You can use this glue effectively in greenhouses, or you can incorporate it on flypaper.

Natural Pesticides

Here are some extremely useful natural pesticides, which can be used in your garden, to deal with pests. The best thing about them is that they are not going to have any harmful side effects. Also, when you use them on the vegetables, these vegetables are going to be totally organic because you have not sprayed them with chemical-based pesticides for pest control.

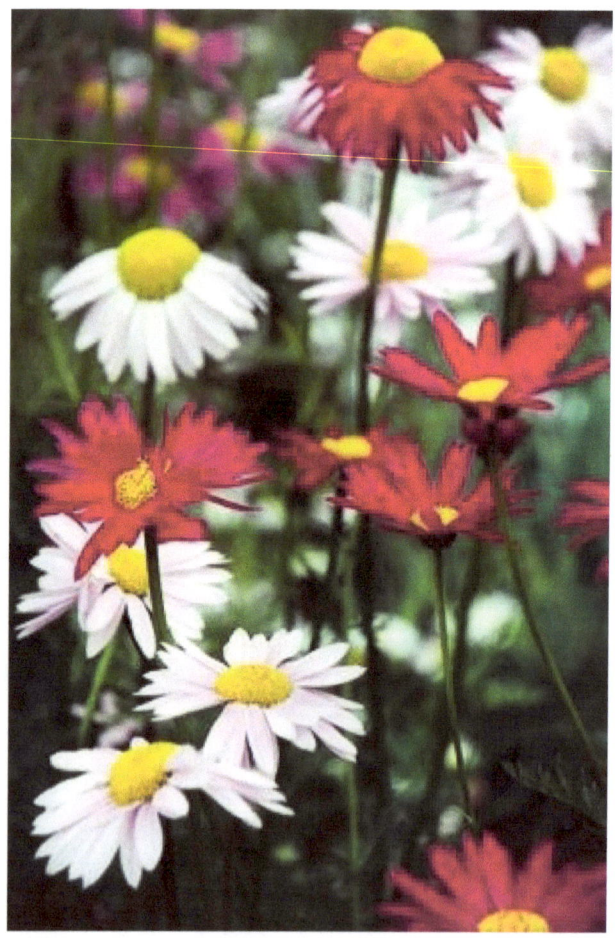

Pyrethrum

Some of these herbs are going to the compost to give you green manure and nourish the soil. Others are going to control pests or act as insecticides, because of the essential oils or insect repellent oils already present in them. For green manure, you can use clover, Lucerne, and alfalfa. For insecticides, you can use Pyrethrum, which are able to control aphids, spider mites, and leaf hoppers.

Quassia – Picraena exelsa – is excellent for controlling thrips, slugs, leaf hoppers, and mealy bugs. In the same manner, at home, all you have to do is leave some cucumber skins on the floor for a couple of nights, and all the pests, including cockroaches are going to disappear. In fact, I saw a gardener doing this in his green house, because he wanted to get rid of wood lice. He also placed some garlic near his roses to get rid of all the aphids. In the same may, if you place garlic and chives near peas and lettuce, you are not going to suffer from aphid attack. In ancient times, hyssop was always grown near beans to prevent black fly and pieces of the hollow stem of Angelica were scattered among all the herbs, so that earwigs could not infest the herbal garden.

Take some white hellebore and chop its root into small pieces. Now scatter these pieces all over the garden and get rid of all the rodents, including mice and rats.

Here is one gardening tip, which he told me has been used extensively down the centuries, even though people have forgotten about it. Compost made at home is excellent as an organic fertilizer, but it can be accelerated really fast with the addition of some herbs which are excellent decomposing material promoters.

So if you want to break the waste down faster, make up a mixture of Valerian, dandelion, chamomile, nettle, yarrow, and bark of the oak in equal quantities. You can use either whole plants, leaves or the bark to form thin layers, interspersed with layer of compost forming green rubbish and soil. Also remember to moisturize this pile with water, as you make it. Compost growth is accelerated, especially in warm weather, so make sure that the box or the compost bin is ventilated adequately.

Animal Care Solutions

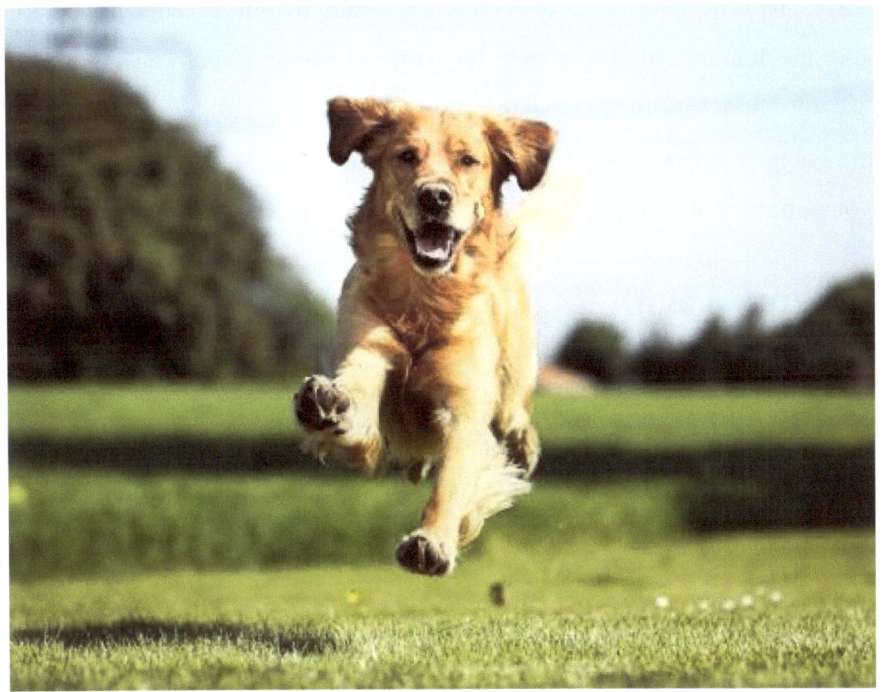

For all of us who like a dog around, one of the major problems of having this animal is that they are regularly infested with lice and fleas. Here is one natural solution to get rid of any sort of insect upon your dog or cat's shiny coat. Just take some walnut leaves and boil them in water until you have a concentrated decoction. You can also use pyrethrum, wormwood, and Derris to make up this decoction. Use this liquid to soak the skin thoroughly, either as a dip or as a wash/lotion. After that, comb the dead insects out of their hair.

Herbal Beauty Products

The ancient Romans like to say that they were the first to throw flowers and leaves in hot water in order to get a scented bath, but this practice has been very much in use in other parts of the world millenniums before Romans began writing history. So here are some natural herbal bath products which are going to help you use herbs effectively and beautifully to cleanse yourself.

Making a Bath Bag

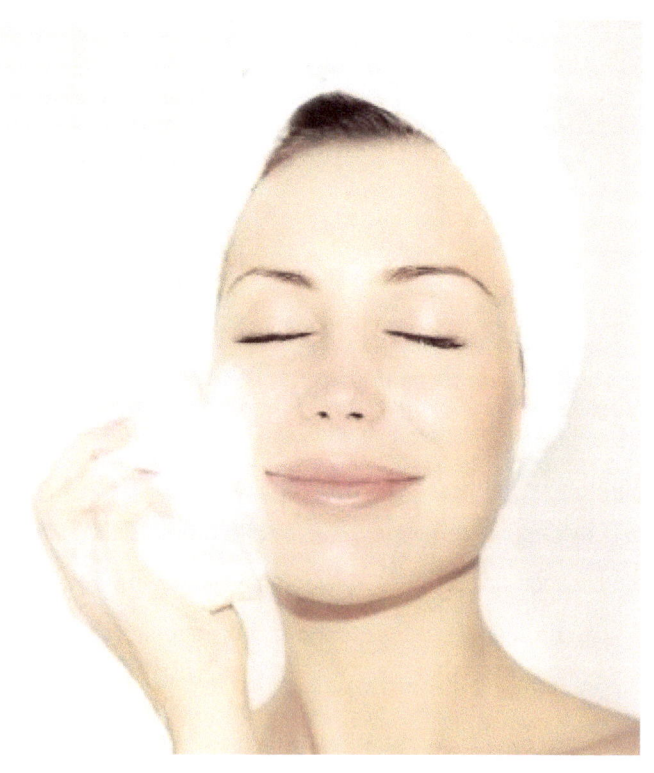

This is easily made by taking up a square of cheesecloth and filling it up with your preferred herbs and oatmeal. This bag should be about 18 x 18 inches and you can tie the corners with 2 feet of ribbon. One cup oatmeal and 2 teaspoons full of your favorite herb is excellent for delicate and sensitive skins. Also, they are capable of curing inflamed and irritated skin conditions. The best thing about oats is that the skin is cleaned and bleached at the same time.

Just wet the bag and use it as a sponge all over the body, washing the skin with the liquid which is seeping through the cloth. The more water you put in the bag, the softer it is going to feel, and the oats are going to remain damp and creamy. After you have finished, you can throw the oats on your compost heap and wash this bath bag. Remember that the proportion of oatmeal is twice that of the herbs used. Stimulating herbs include bay, fennel, lavender, basil, mint, pine, rosemary, sage, fennel, and thyme. The relaxing herbs include Jasmine, chamomile, catnip, vervain, and lime flowers.

Healing herbs are marigold, comfrey, mint, and yarrow. I use marigold water – washed and cleaned marigold petals boiling water, and then filtered as an excellent antiseptic.

How to Make Your Own Bath Oil

The problem with essential oils is that the moment you put them in water, they are not going to mix properly. Apart from that, you may find yourself quite shiny with oil, when you come out of the bath. In order to prevent this, take half a cup of castor oil –this oil is excellent for your hair. It is also excellent for making your bathwater oil. To this half cup of castor oil, you are going to add just 10 drops of your favorite essential oil like lavender oil, rosemary, sandalwood, or pine. Put this in a glass bottle after you have shaken it thoroughly, and just one teaspoonful in your bathwater is going to give you excellently perfumed bath oil.

You can also use an aromatic oil, but remember that these are already powerful, and as they are more powerful and concentrated than essential oils, using them in in your bath oil, may give you a headache. So try using just about 1 – 2 drops at the time in half a cup, to see whether the aroma relaxes you or gives you a raging headache.

Making Your Own Bath Salts

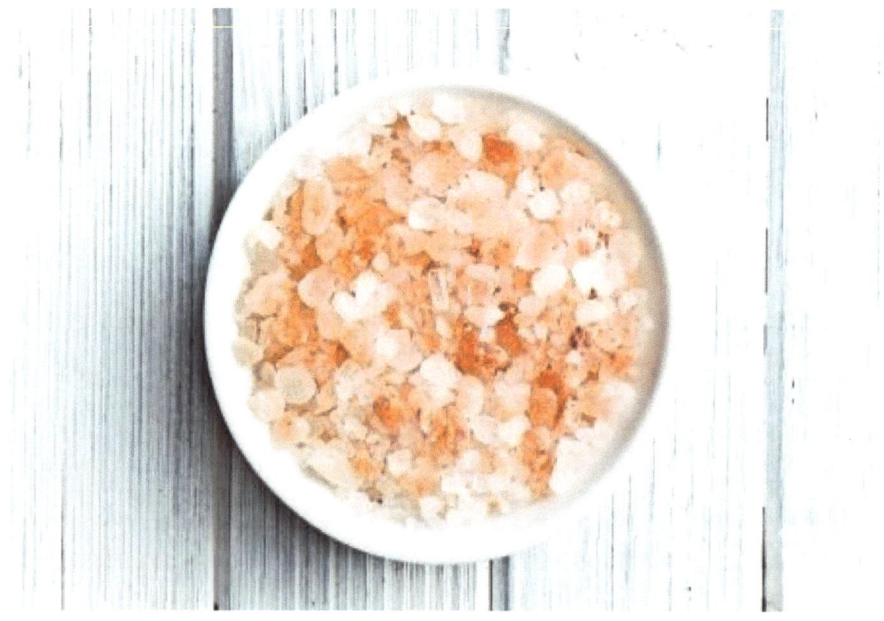

Just a handful of bath salts – I like the ones that sizzle and fizz, somewhat like soda bicarbonate – it is soda bicarbonate! – are capable of making a boring bath, something like a spa experience. That is because the soda base of these salts is capable of neutralizing the acid factor of the skin and that is why the perfume clings to your skin. So what you need is 140 grams of soda bicarbonate, 80 – 85 g of Orris powdered root, and a few drops of your favorite essential oils, like rosemary, lavender, geranium, bergamot, or Neroli.

Mix them together in a pestle and mortar. Why I do not use the 21st century way of just putting them in a blender and allowing to blend, is that I get plenty of my bad temper out in just beating the bejabbers out of these helpless unsuspecting ingredients, while mixing the essential oils thoroughly.

Once you put them in a glass bottle, these are going to keep for about 3 months, as long as the container is air tight.

Making Traditional Soap Balls

Traditional soap was originally made with olive oil, animal fats, and lye. Even today, I can get it in the local market to wash my clothes!

Once I asked a French friend of mine, why in the medieval times, people in Europe were afraid of taking baths, and she said the tradition was *L'eau abime le peau* – or water destroys the skin! Actually, it was not the water which destroyed the skin, but the cleansing soap which was used, which was full of caustic soda – lye. Just imagine yourself rubbing yourself with caustic soda and then going into water. It was only the very rich who could afford soap of Castile.

Here is one way traditional soap was made, as a base. It was grated and then essential oils, powdered roots, leaves, and petals added to the mixture, especially in Italy and France. So you can adapt the medieval recipe to your own requirements, and we are lucky that we can find these ingredients commonly in the market today. The recipe written in 21st century from the original document is going to read somewhat like this. These people knew nothing about punctuation, so there are no ye grande olde full stoppes!

"Take a pound of a fine white Castile soap, shave it thin into a pint of rosewater, and let it stand for 2 – 3 days than pour out the water from it and put it into half a pint of fresh water and let it stand for one whole day, then pour out that and put half a pint more and let it be for one night more than put half an ounce of powder called sweet marjoram, a quarter of an ounce of powder of winter savory leaves, 2 or 3 drops of oil of Spike, and the oil of cloves, 3 grains of musk and as much ambergris, work all together in a mortar, with the powder of an almond cake, dried and beaten as small as fine flour, so roll it around in your hands in rosewater. "

If you do not have an almond cake, you can use a macaroon or a ratafia biscuit. Whew!

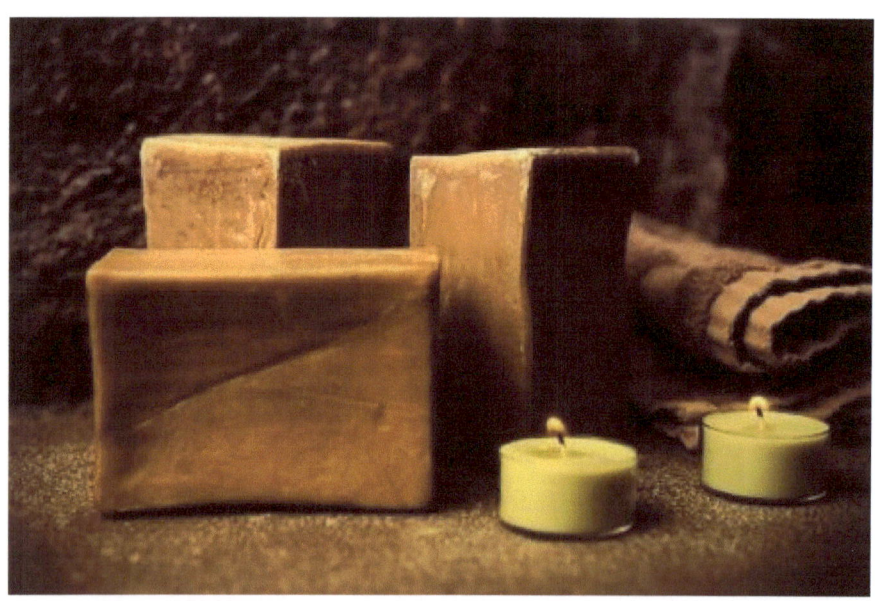

Aleppo soap, made with olive oil and lye

The easiest modern version is going to take a large bar of simple soap, ¼ cup of rosewater, and 3 drops of lavender essential oil. Do the grating of the bar of soap into the rosewater; allow it to stand in the liquid for about 15 minutes before you blend it completely in a blender. Now keep adding the oil of lavender a drop at a time during the blending process.

Once it has blended softly and smoothly, pour the mixture into a basin and allow it to stand for a day or so. After that, you are going to form into small bath balls, by breaking off pieces and rolling them between your palms. Allow them to dry. For a smooth and attractive finish, you can dip your hands in rosewater when you are doing the rolling.

Natural Body Powders

A little bit of talcum is always welcome and that is why hydrated magnesium silicate known as "talk" in Persian has been used as a bath powder for centuries. It reached Europe in the 16th century and became an integral part of European toiletry. It was slightly greasy to the touch. But the powder that you are getting in the market today is a mixture of corn flour, calcium carbonate, and other filling substances with a little bit of perfume added to it.

The original recipe for Poudre a la Mousseline (Poodr a laa moos-leen) is made up of 450 g base, 170 g of powdered coriander seeds, 50 g of powdered mace, 25 g of powdered cloves, 25 g of powdered sandalwood, and Cassia/cinnamon and the herbal bases made of 60% orris root, 30% cornstarch, and 10 percent rice flour. Blend all of these together, and do a little bit of experimentation on your own skin to see which proportion suits you the best.

Foot Care Talcum Powder

Just take one tablespoonful of cornstarch, one teaspoonful of bicarbonate of soda, a few drops of peppermint extract, half a teaspoon of finely powdered thyme, a few drops of rubbing alcohol, and grind them all together. If you are suffering from athlete's foot, especially between the toes, be sure to add some lemon peel, so that the oil can cure the fungus. After that, you can dust the area with this talcum powder.

Natural Anti-wrinkle Lotion

This is a Middle Eastern ancient recipe where poppies grew in abundance. Take 15 – 20 petals of the poppy, and drop them into 280 g of boiling water. Allow to infuse for 20 minutes, and then filter. Use this morning and night to get rid of any sort of wrinkles.

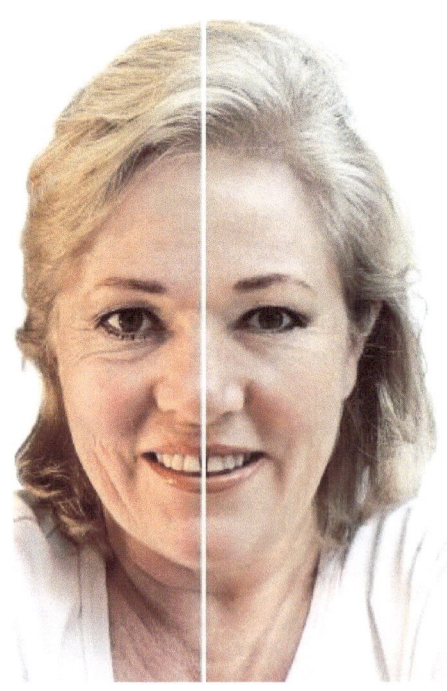

Rosemary and Herbal Infusion for Haircare

It has been said that if you have rosemary in your garden, you are never going to suffer from any sort of hair problems. Rosemary has been known since ancient times to protect your hair, and keep it healthy, and shiny. Just make an infusion of rosemary leaves, if you are a brunette, and chamomile leaves and flower or nettle leaves, if you are blonde, if you are auburn or brown haired. 560 mL of water is going to do to every 25 g weight of herb. Boil this water. Place the herbs in a suitable container like a basin or a jug and then pour the boiling water over them. Allow them to steep for 30 minutes before you filter them with cheesecloth. Allow this infusion to cool down and mix it with your regular shampoo. You do not need any conditioning after you have washed your hair in the normal manner.

Natural Hair Rinses

You can consider them as scalp and hair conditioners, one may use vinegar and beer, lemon, white wine, or cider vinegar as the last rinse, after you have used your shampoo. Just add one teaspoonful to the last of your rinse water. You can also steep rosemary spikes in boiling water for half an hour. After that, strain cool, filter, and use whenever necessary. Thus it is not surprising that rosemary is one of the most important ingredients in the multibillion dollar head and hair care industry.

Apart from this, I am going to suggest another natural haircare rinse which may be something you are using under an expensive brand-name. It is made up of equal parts of chamomile, fennel, rosemary, sage, nettle, lime, flowers, horsetail, and yarrow. All of them are added to water, infused, filtered, and bottled. If you have blonde hair, you are going to add more chamomile. If you have darker hair, you are going to add more rosemary.

Placed 25 g of these herbs into a jug and pour 560 mL of boiling water over them, steep until they are cool, then strain and filter. In the general use this as a final rinse for general health and luster to your hair.

If you want to condition your hair with a massage, add equal quantities of fennel, chamomile, yarrow, and nettle in 560 mL of sunflower oil. I put them all in coconut oil, and the results were excellent. Put them all in sunlight, in a glass bottle, and allow to cool so that the essential oils are released and infused in the base oil.

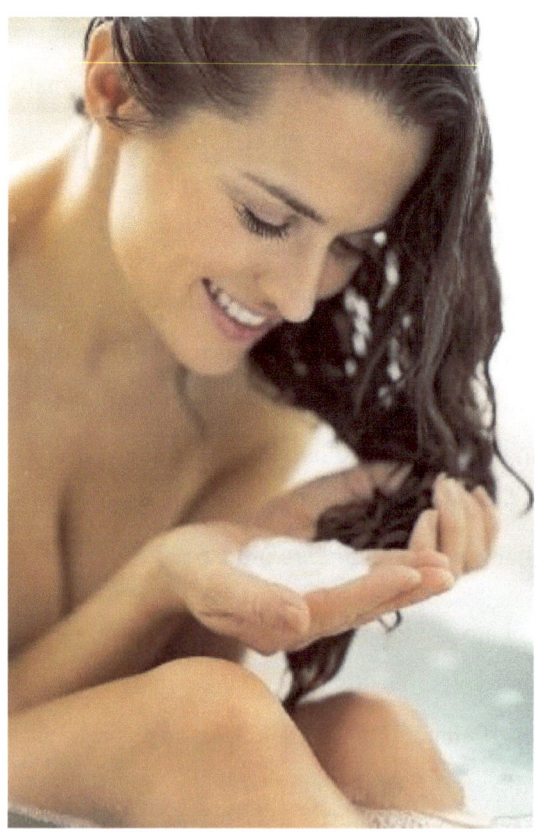

Conclusion

The use of herbs for beneficial purposes is so vast that it is going to take a couple of lifetimes in order to collect them. Apart from this, think of all the knowledge that has been lost on the ages, and is still being discovered everyday.

This book has given you some information on how you can use these herbs domestically, and with some cosmetic recipes. This information and knowledge is accurate in keeping with our other herbal books, in our learning series.

So take full benefit of this book, save some money by making your own herbal products, Live Long and Prosper!

Author Bio

Dueep Jyot Singh is a Management and IT Professional who managed to gather Postgraduate qualifications in Management and English and Degrees in Science, French and Education while pursuing different enjoyable career options like being an hospital administrator, IT,SEO and HRD Database Manager/ trainer, movie , radio and TV scriptwriter, theatre artiste and public speaker, lecturer in French, Marketing and Advertising, ex-Editor of Hearts On Fire (now known as Solstice) Books Missouri USA, advice columnist and cartoonist, publisher and Aviation School trainer, ex-moderator on Medico.in, banker, student councilor ,travelogue writer … among other things!

One fine morning, she decided that she had enough of killing herself by Degrees and went back to her first love -- writing. It's more enjoyable! She already has 48 published academic and 14 fiction- in- different- genre books under her belt.

When she is not designing websites or making Graphic design illustrations for clients , she is browsing through old bookshops hunting for treasures, of which she has an enviable collection – including R.L. Stevenson, O.Henry, Dornford Yates, Maurice Walsh, De Maupassant, Victor Hugo, Sapper, C.N. Williamson, "Bartimeus" and the crown of her collection- Dickens "The Old Curiosity Shop," and "Martin Chuzzlewit" and so on… Just call her "Renaissance Woman" - collecting herbal remedies, acting like Universal Helping Hand/Agony Aunt, or escaping to her dear mountains for a bit of exploring, collecting herbs and plants, and trekking.

Check out some of the other JD-Biz Publishing books

Gardening Series on Amazon

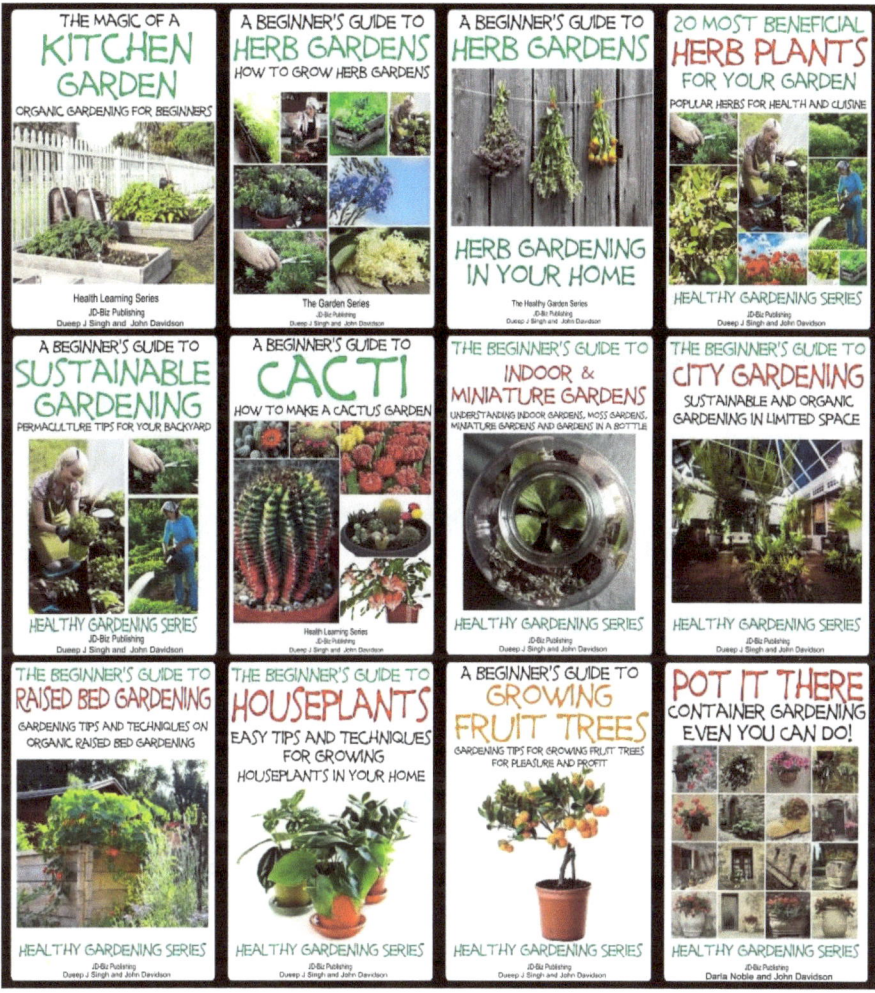

Download Free Books!

http://MendonCottageBooks.com

Health Learning Series

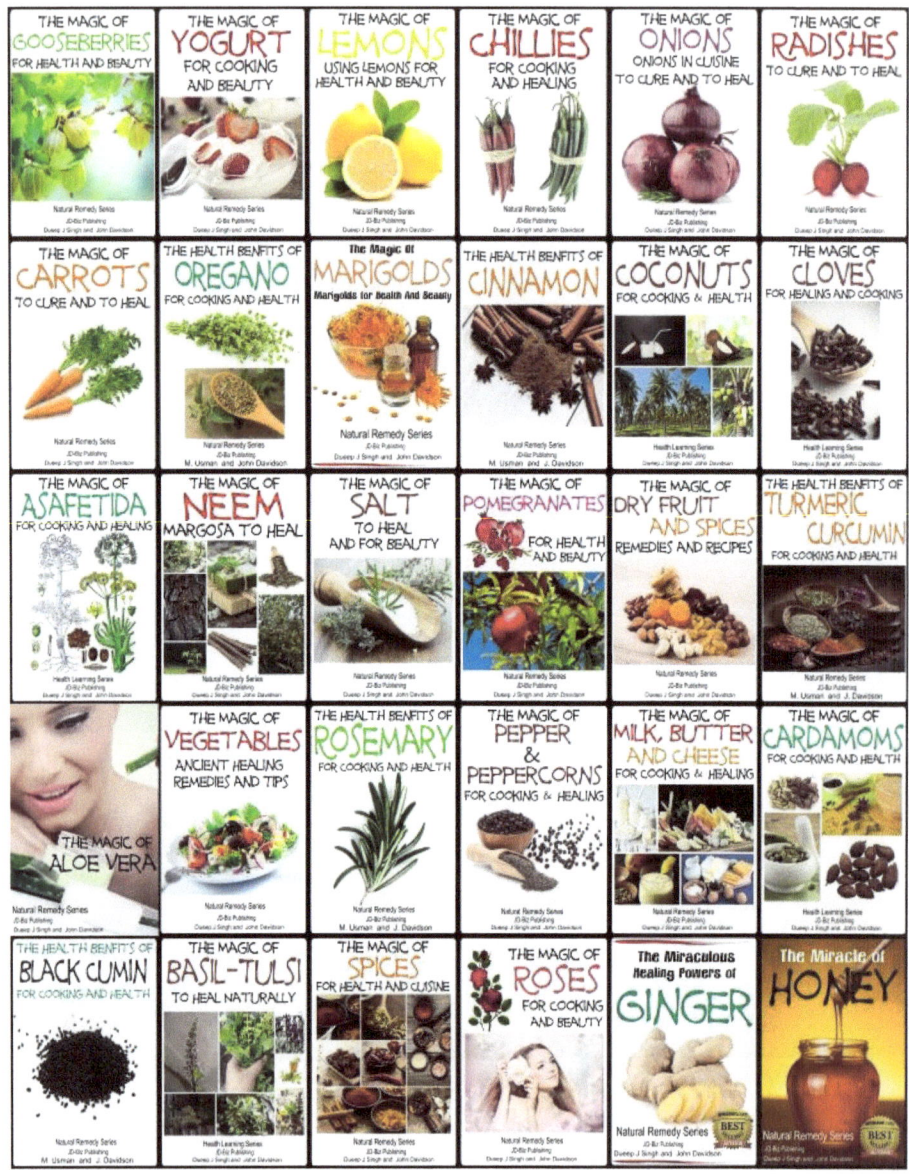

Country Life Books

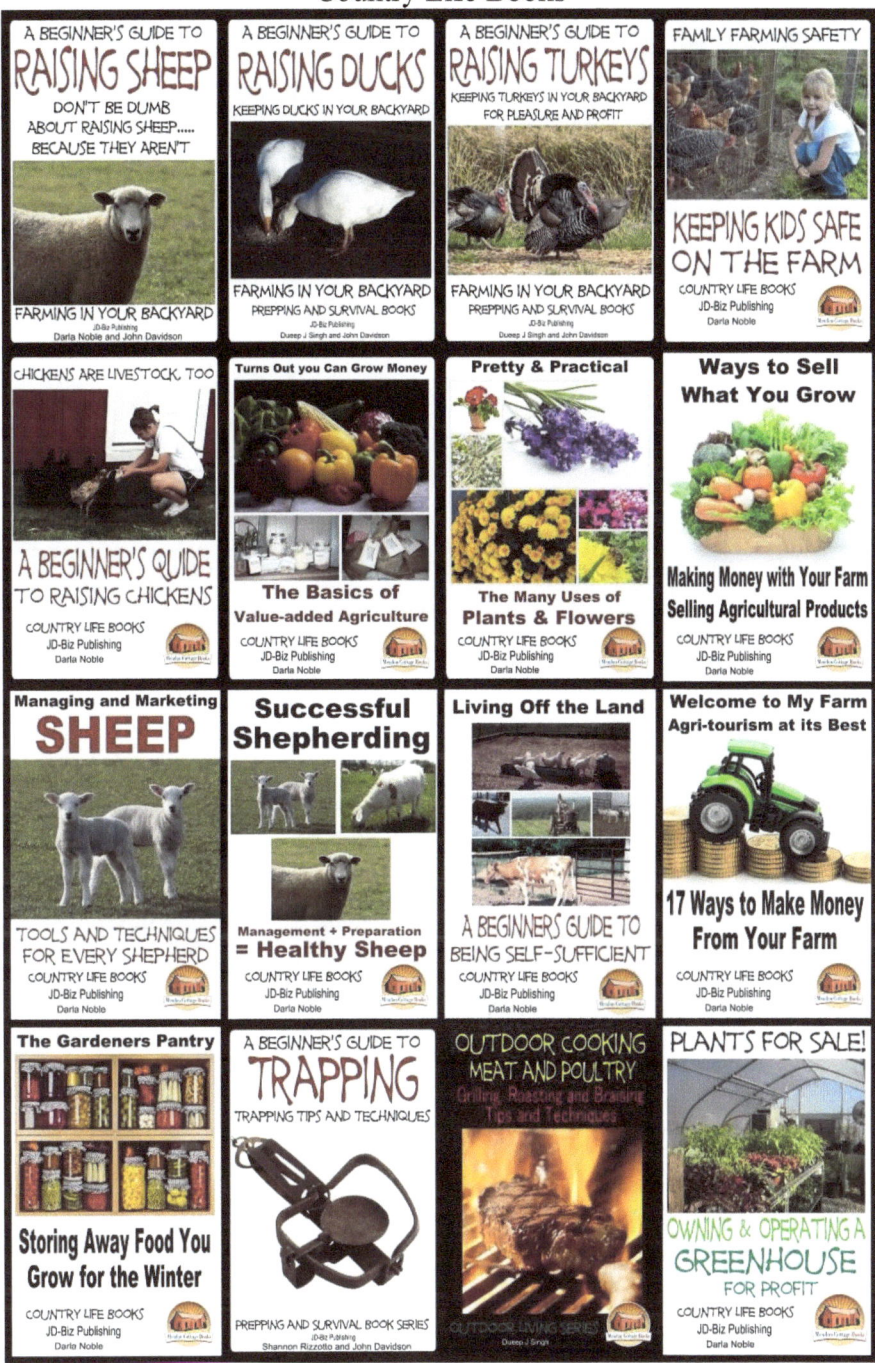

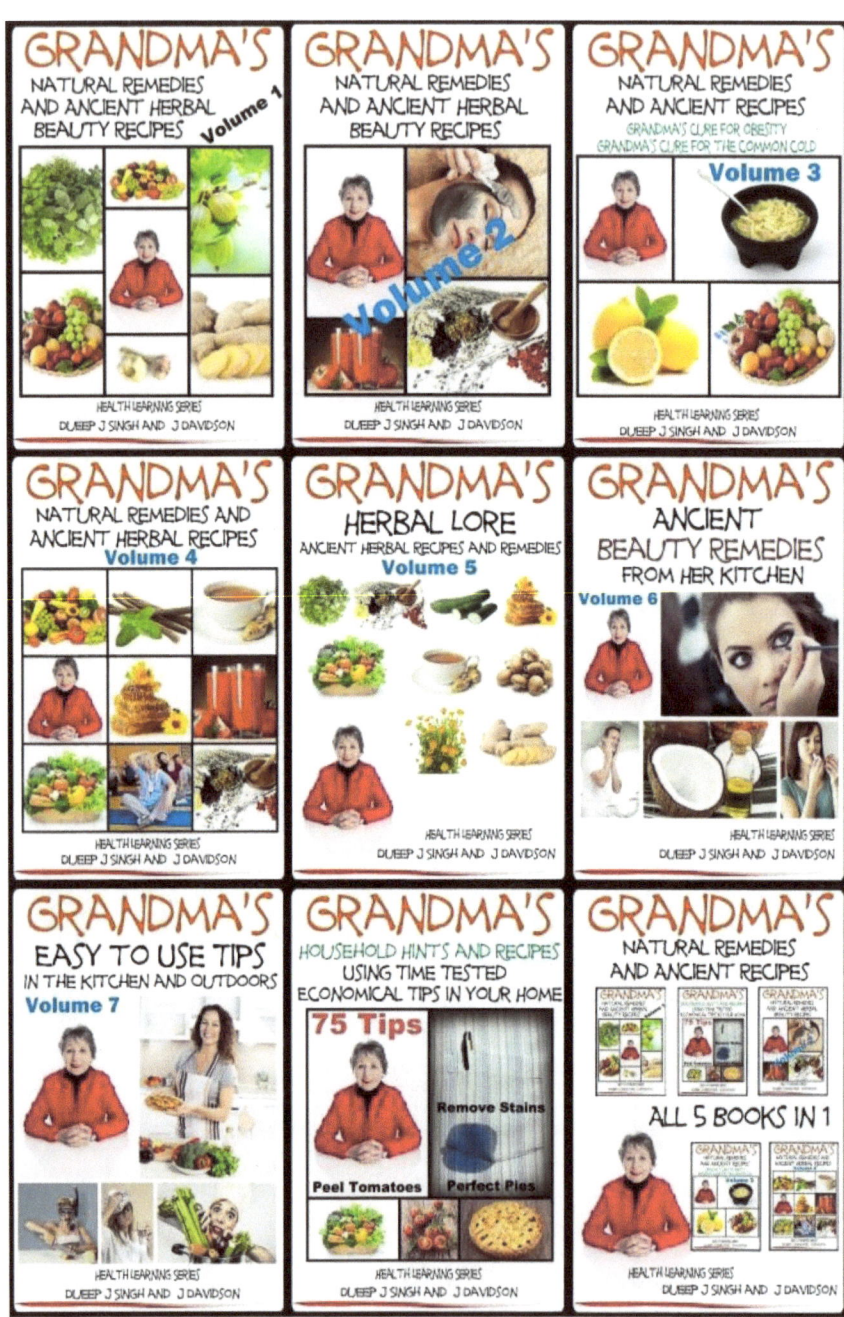

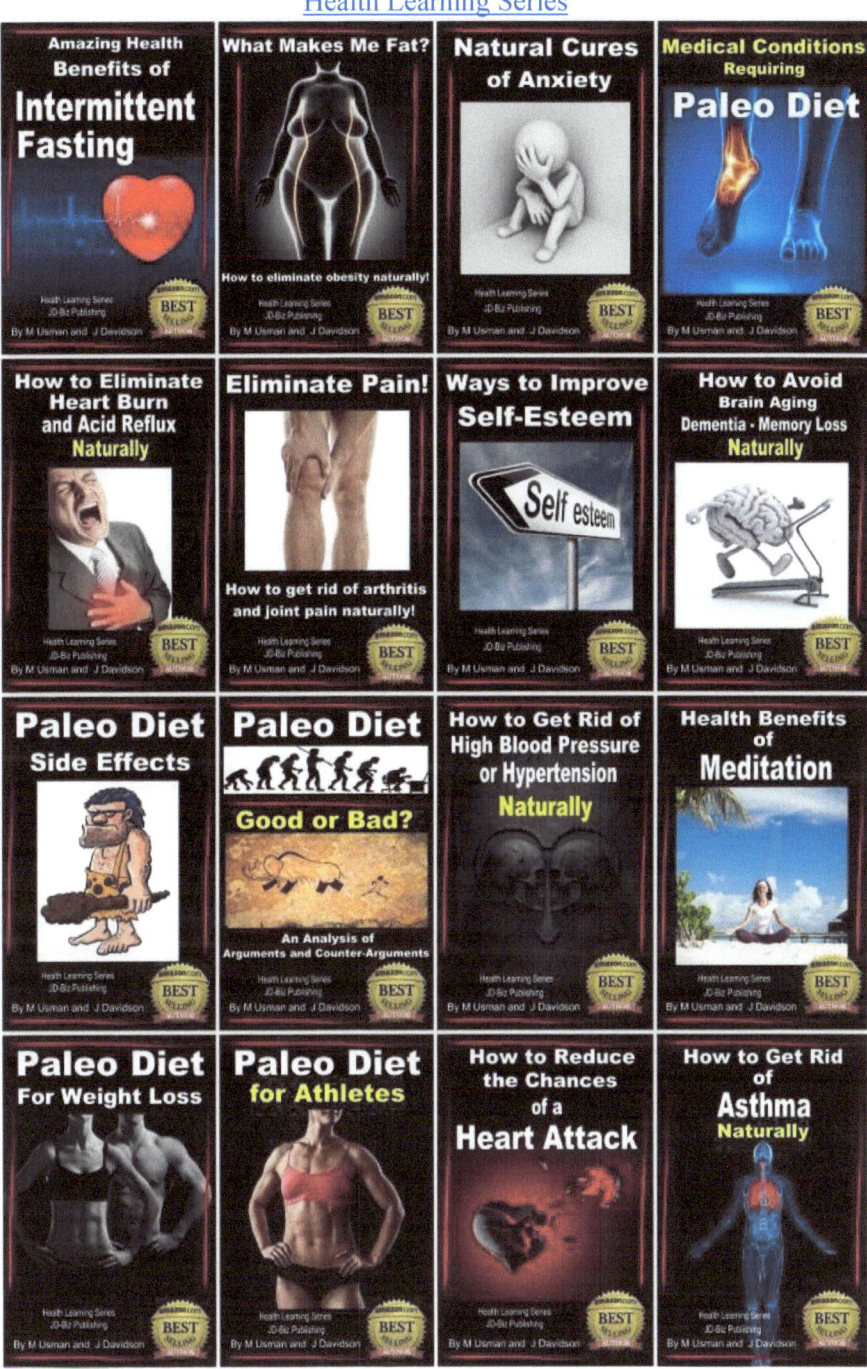

Amazing Animal Book Series

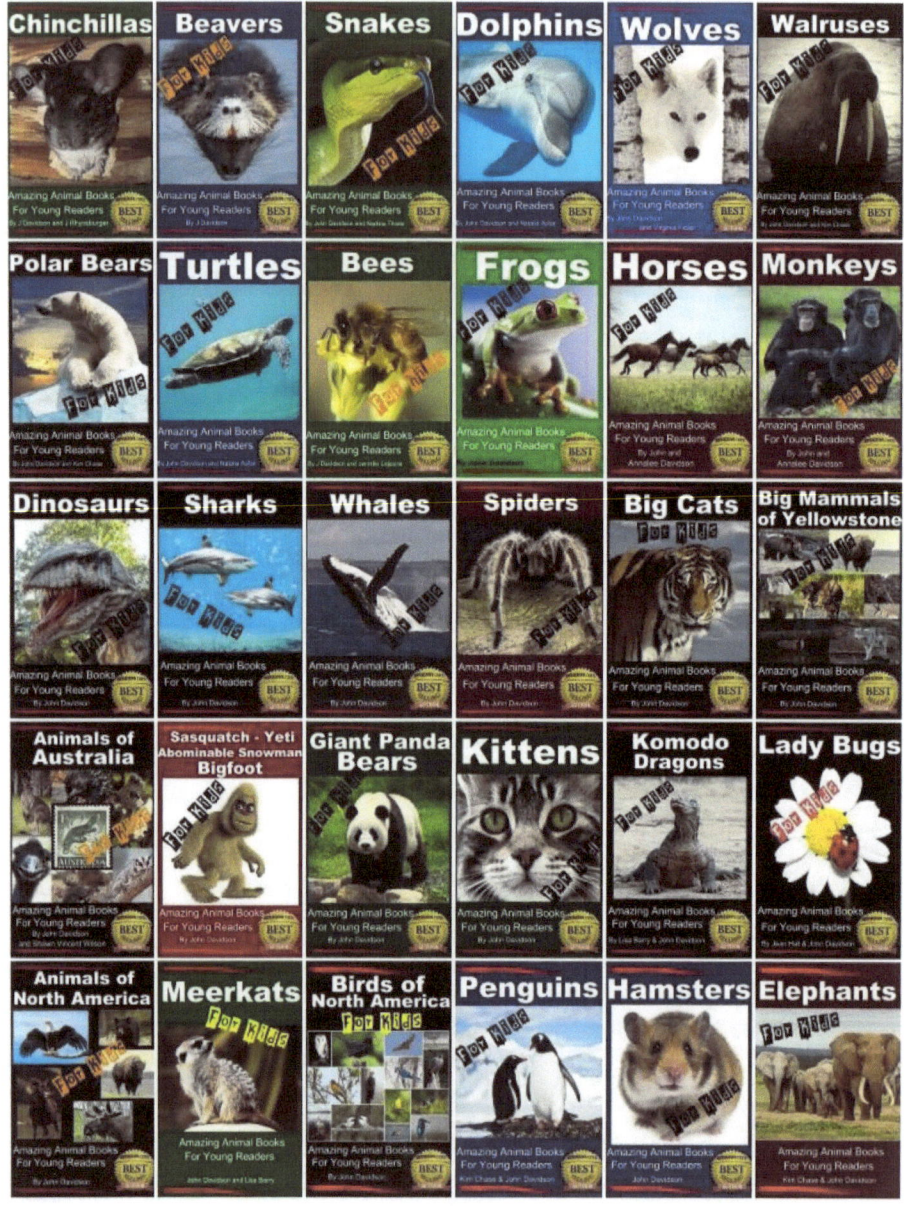

Learn To Draw Series

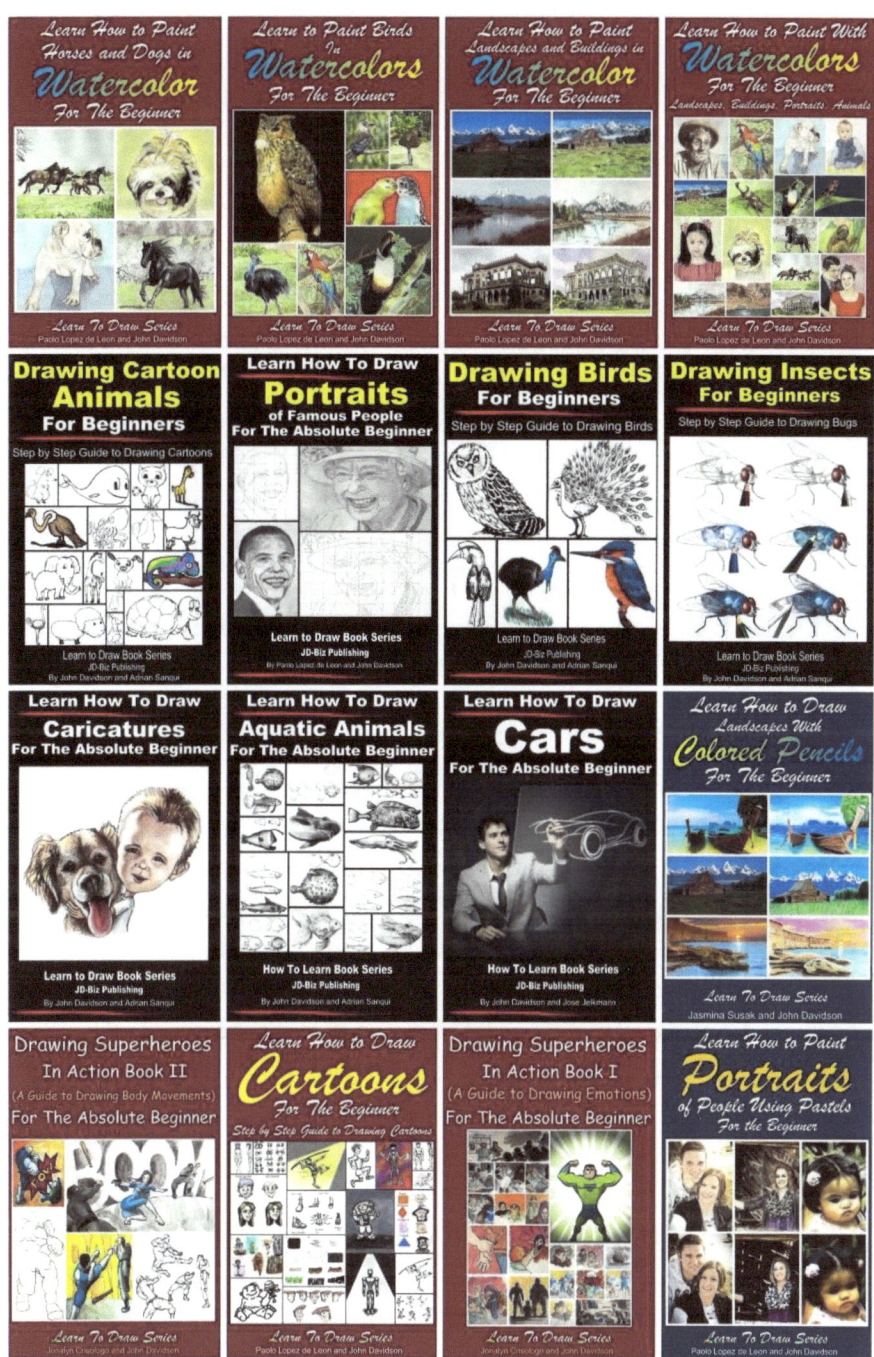

How to Build and Plan Books

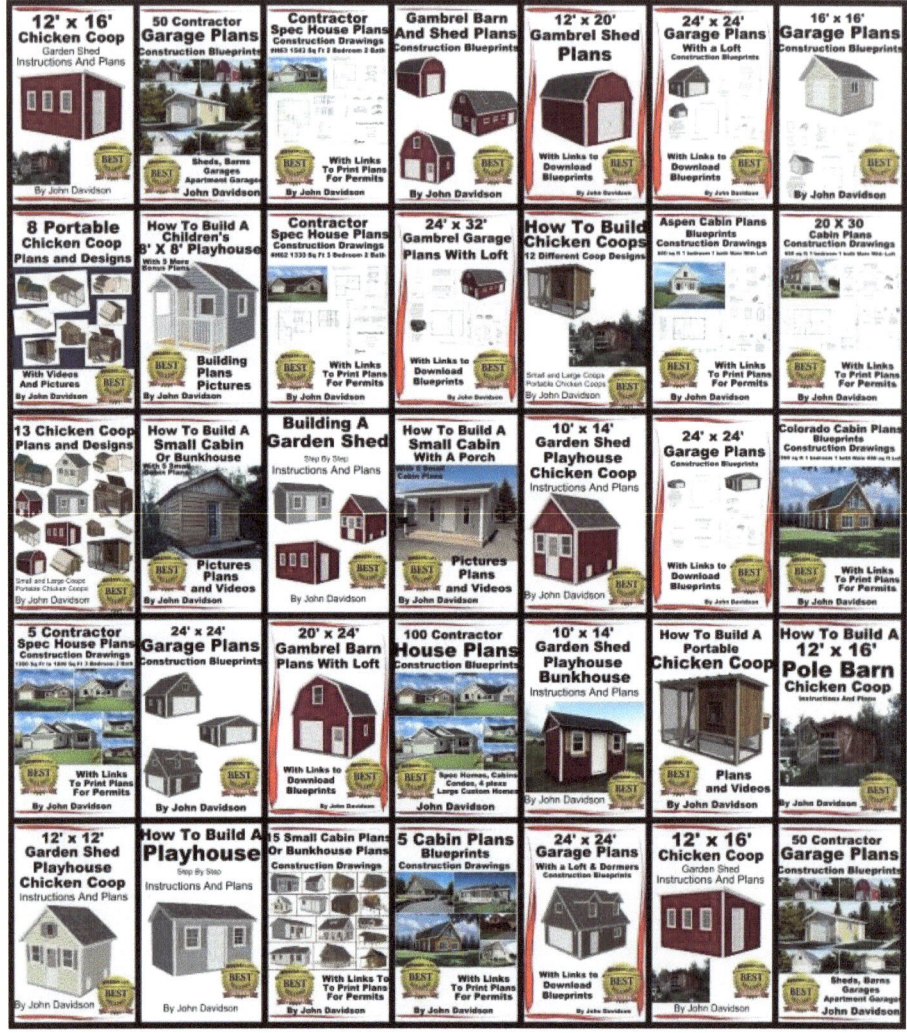

Entrepreneur Book Series

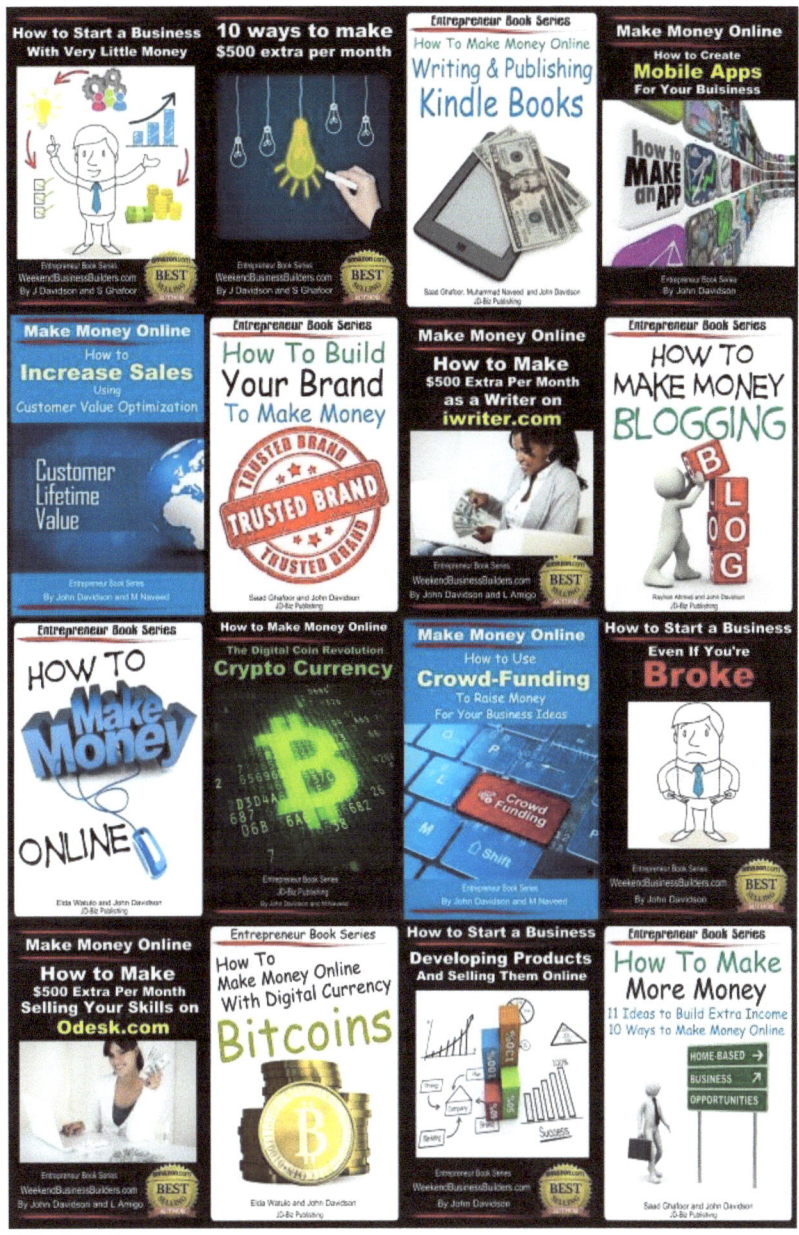

Our books are available at

1. Amazon.com

2. Barnes and Noble

3. Itunes

4. Kobo

5. Smashwords

6. Google Play Books

Download Free Books!

http://MendonCottageBooks.com

Publisher

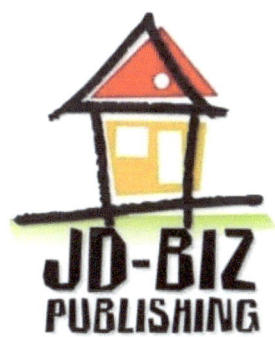

JD-Biz Corp

P O Box 374

Mendon, Utah 84325

http://www.jd-biz.com/

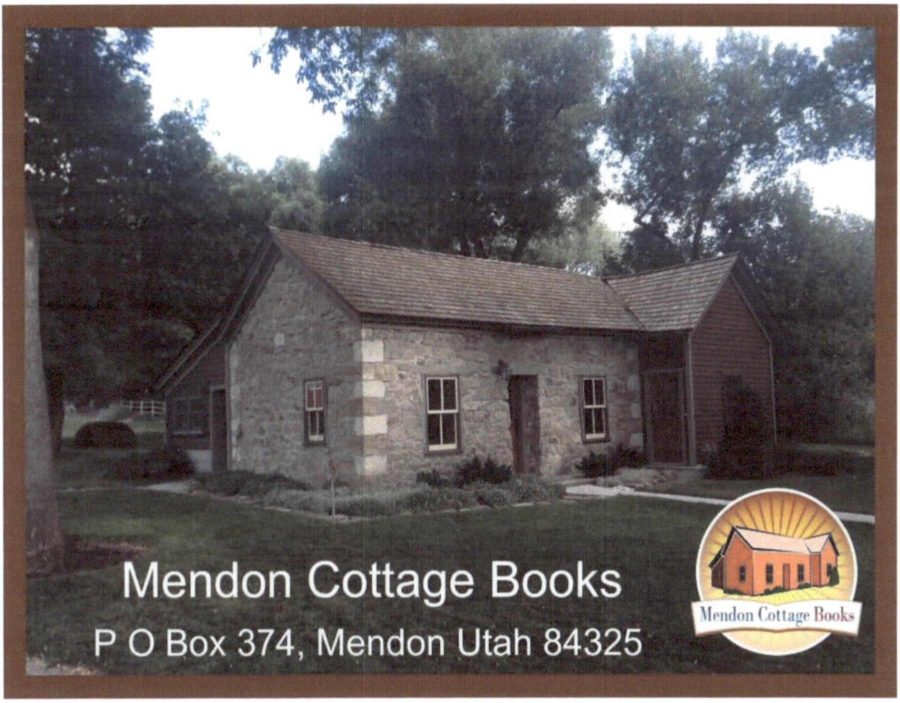

Mendon Cottage Books

P O Box 374, Mendon Utah 84325

www.ingramcontent.com/pod-product-compliance
Lightning Source LLC
Chambersburg PA
CBHW050829290526
45792CB00001B/325